The Complete Air Fryer Lean And Green & Smoothie Cookbook

Healthy And Tasty Dishes & Smoothie Recipes To Stay In Shape

Alan Green

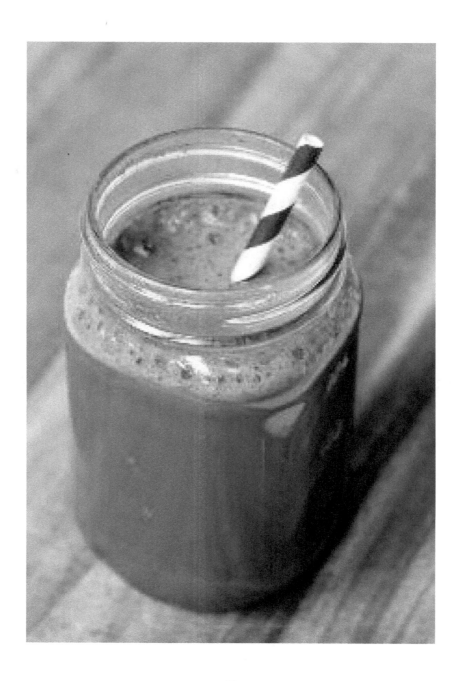

Table of contents

Air Fryer Green Beans

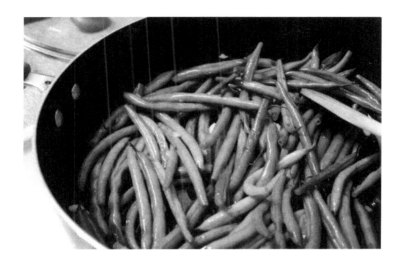

Prep Time: 5 mins

Cook Time: 10 mins

Total Time: 15 mins

Ingredients

1 lb green beans

1 tbsp olive oil

1/2 tsp salt

1/4 tsp pepper

Instructions

Trim the green beans, then toss with olive oil, salt, and pepper.

Put prepared green beans in the air fryer basket and cook at 400F for 10 minutes, shaking the basket halfway through.

Nutrition

Calories: 66kcal | Carbohydrates: 8g | Protein: 2g | Fat: 4g | Saturated Fat: 1g | Sodium: 298mg | Potassium: 239mg | Fiber: 3g | Sugar: 4g | Vitamin A: 782IU | Vitamin C: 14mg | Calcium: 42mg | Iron: 1mg

Healthy Air Fryer Chicken and Veggies (20 Minutes!)

Prep Time: 5 minutes

Cook Time: 15 minutes

Total Time: 20 minutes

Ingredients

1 pound chicken breast, chopped into bite-size pieces (2-3 medium chicken breasts)

1 cup broccoli florets (fresh or frozen)

1 zucchini chopped

1 cup bell pepper chopped (any colors you like)

1/2 onion chopped

2 cloves garlic minced or crushed

2 tablespoons olive oil

1/2 teaspoon EACH garlic powder, chili powder, salt, pepper 1 tablespoon Italian seasoning (or spice blend of choice)

Instructions

Preheat air fryer to 400F.

Chop the veggies and chicken into small bite-size pieces and transfer to a large mixing bowl.

Add the oil and seasoning to the bowl and toss to combine.

Add the chicken and veggies to the preheated air fryer and cook for 10 minutes, shaking halfway, or until the chicken and veggies are charred and chicken is cooked through. If your air fryer is small, you may have to cook them in 2-3 batches.

Nutrition

Serving: 1serving | Calories: 230kcal | Carbohydrates: 8g | Protein: 26g | Fat: 10g | Saturated Fat: 2g | Cholesterol: 73mg | Sodium: 437mg | Potassium: 734mg | Fiber: 3g | Sugar: 4g | Vitamin A: 1584IU | Vitamin C: 79mg | Calcium: 50mg | Iron: 1mg

Fried Green Beans (Air Fryer)

Prep Time: 5 minutes

Cook Time: 5 minutes

Total Time: 10 minutes

Ingredients

1 lb. fresh green beans (cleaned and trimmed)

1 tsp. oil

1/4 tsp. garlic powder

1/8 tsp. sea salt

Instructions

Toss all the Ingredients together in a bowl to coat the green beans with oil and spices.

Transfer about half of the green beans to the air fryer basket. (You'll have to do this in two batches or the beans won't cook properly) Spread them out as evenly as possible and return the basket to the air fryer.

Adjust temp to 400 and set time to 5 minutes, or whichever time you chose from the chart above, and press start.

When done, remove the basket from the fryer and turn the beans out onto a platter (repeat with the second half of the beans).

If you try the beans and they aren't cooked enough to your liking, simply return them to the air fryer in the basket and cook in 2-minute increments until they are cooked to your liking. Cool slightly and serve.

Nutrition

Serving: 0.25the recipe | Calories: 47kcal | Carbohydrates: 8g | Protein: 2g | Fat: 1g | Saturated Fat: 1g | Sodium: 67mg | Potassium: 239mg | Fiber: 3g | Sugar: 4g | Vitamin A: 782IU | Vitamin C: 14mg | Calcium: 42mg | Iron: 1mg

Air Fryer Green Beans

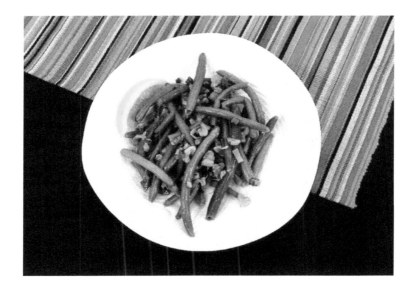

Prep Time: 5 mins

Cook Time: 15 mins

Total Time: 20 mins

Ingredients

1 pound (454 g) fresh green beans, ends trimmed and halved

1-2 tablespoons (15 ml) olive oil or spray

1/2 teaspoon (2.5 ml) garlic powder

Salt and pepper, to taste

Fresh lemon slices

Instructions

In a bowl, combine green beans, oil, garlic powder, salt, and pepper. Place the seasoned green beans in an air fryer basket.

Air Fry 360°F for about 10-14 minutes depending on your preferred doneness. Toss and shake about 2 times during cooking.

Season with salt and pepper, to taste. Serve with lemon slices or wedges

Nutrition

Calories: 67kcal | Carbohydrates: 8g | Protein: 2g | Fat: 4g | Saturated Fat: 1g | Sodium: 7mg | Potassium: 239mg | Fiber: 3g | Sugar: 4g | Vitamin A: 782IU | Vitamin C: 14mg | Calcium: 42mg | Iron: 1mg

Air Fryer Stuffed Peppers

Prep Time: 15 Minutes

Cook Time: 15 Minutes

Total Time: 30 Minutes

Ingredients

6 Green Bell Peppers

1 Lb Lean Ground Beef

1 Tbsp Olive Oil

1/4 Cup Green Onion Diced

1/4 Cup Fresh Parsley

1/2 Tsp Ground Sage

1/2 Tsp Garlic Salt

1 Cup Cooked Rice

1 Cup Marinara Sauce More to Taste

1/4 Cup Shredded Mozzarella Cheese

Instructions

Warm-up a medium-sized skillet with the ground beef and cook until well done.

Drain the beef and return to the pan.

Add in the olive oil, green onion, parsley, sage, and salt. Mix this well.

Add in the cooked rice and marinara, mix well.

Cut the top off of each pepper and clean the seeds out.

Scoop the mixture into each of the peppers and place it in the basket of the air fryer. (I did 4 the first round, 2 the second to make them fit.)

Cook for 10 minutes at 355*, carefully open and add cheese.

Cook for an additional 5 minutes or until peppers are slightly soft and cheese is melted.

Serve.

Nutrition Information

Calories: 296| Total Fat: 13g| Saturated Fat: 4g| Trans Fat: 0g| Unsaturated Fat: 7g| Cholesterol: 70mg| Sodium: 419mg| Carbohydrates: 19g| Fiber: 2g| Sugar: 6g| Protein: 25g

Air Fryer Weight Watchers Stuffed Peppers

Prep Time: 5 Mins

Cook Time: 25 Mins

Total Time: 30 Mins

Ingredients

6 bell peppers red, yellow, and orange

1/4 cup water

1/2 lb ground turkey breast LEAN

1 small zucchini small dice

2 cups crushed tomatoes no salt added

1 cup mushrooms small dice

1.5 cups cauliflower rice

1 tbsp Worcestershire sauce

1 tsp salt

3 Babybel Mini Light Cheese Rounds grated

Instructions

Heat non-stick skillet on medium-high

Add water, ground turkey, zucchini, and mushrooms

Brown for five minutes and add salt

While turkey is browning, heat cauliflower rice in microwave according to package directions To the turkey, add Worcestershire, rice, and tomatoes and simmer for 2-3 minutes

While turkey mixture is cooking, prep peppers by slicing off tops and clean the insides (save the pepper tops to use in other recipes)

Spoon turkey mixture into peppers

Air Fryer Instructions: AF at 350 for 10 minutes. Open AF and add shredded cheese. Air Fry 5 minutes more until cheese melts and browns

Oven Instructions: Cover with foil and bake at 350 for 30 minutes. Uncover and add shredded cheese. Bake an additional 15 minutes (uncovered)

Nutrition Value

Calories: 400kcal, Carbohydrates: 27g, Protein: 66.1g, Fat: 4.4g, Saturated Fat: 1.3g, Cholesterol: 146mg, Sodium: 1118mg, Potassium: 520mg, Fiber: 7.4g, Sugar: 18g, Calcium: 211mg, Iron: 3mg

Easy Air Fryer Parmesan-Crusted Tilapia

Prep Time: 3 Mins

Cook Time: 7 Mins

Total Time: 10 Mins

Ingredients

2 thin tilapia fillets (about 4 ounces) fresh or frozen (times given for both below)

Olive oil pump spray not aerosol or 1 tablespoon olive oil

1/4 teaspoon salt

1/4 teaspoon ground pepper (optional)

2 tablespoons grated Parmesan cheese

1/2 cup fine dry breadcrumbs

Instructions

Place the frozen tilapia fillets on an aluminum or stainless steel baking pan while preheating the air fryer and measuring ingredients.

Crazy Good Tip: These few minutes on the baking pan will ever so slightly thaw the fillets just enough to allow the breadcrumbs to stick to the oil on them. Preheat the air fryer to 390-400 degrees for 3 minutes. Most air fryers preset "air fryer" button is 390F to 400F degrees.

Spray or coat fish fillets with olive oil sprayer or mister or brush with olive oil. (Not Pam aerosol vegetable cooking spray)

Sprinkle both sides of fillets with salt and if desired, pepper.

Sprinkle the top side of fillets with Parmesan cheese.

Place the dry breadcrumbs on a plate and gently press the fish into the breadcrumbs to coat them. If you have trouble getting the breadcrumbs to stick to the fish, wait just a few minutes or

I like to spray the breaded fish again on top with a little bit of olive oil spray (again, not aerosol)

Frozen fish: Air Fry at 390-400 degrees for 9 to 11 minutes, without turning, depending on the thickness of fish until fish flakes easily in the center.

Fresh fish: Air Fry at 390-400 degrees for 7 minutes, without turning, depending on the thickness of fish until fish flakes easily in the center.

Carefully remove the fish with a silicone-coated spatula to prevent scraping the nonstick surface.

Nutrition Value

Calories: 206kcal

Air Fryer Steak Bites & Mushrooms

Prep Time: 10 mins

Cook Time: 18 mins

Total Time: 28 mins

Ingredients

1 lb. (454 g) steaks, cut into 1/2" cubes (ribeye, sirloin, tri-tip, or what you prefer)

8 oz. (227 g) mushrooms (cleaned, washed, and halved)

2 tablespoons (30 ml) butter, melted (or olive oil)

1 teaspoon (5 ml) worcestershire sauce

1/2 teaspoon (2.5 ml) garlic powder, optional

Flakey salt, to taste

Fresh cracked black pepper, to taste

Minced parsley, garnish

Melted butter, for finishing - optional

Chili flakes, for finishing - optional

Instructions

Rinse and thoroughly pat dry the steak cubes. Combine the steak cubes and mushrooms. Coat with the melted butter and then season with Worcestershire sauce, optional garlic powder, and a generous seasoning of salt and pepper.

Preheat the Air Fryer at 400°F for 4 minutes.

Spread the steak and mushrooms in an even layer in the air fryer basket. Air fry at 400°F for 10-18 minutes, shaking and flipping and the steak and mushrooms 2 times through the cooking process (time depends on your preferred doneness, the thickness of the steak, size of air fryer).

Check the steak to see how well done it is cooked. If you want the steak more done, add an extra 2-5 minutes of cooking time.

Garnish with parsley and drizzle with optional melted butter and/or optional chili flakes. Season with additional salt & pepper if desired. Serve warm.

Nutrition Value

Calories: 401kcal | Carbohydrates: 3g | Protein: 32g | Fat: 29g | Saturated Fat: 14g | Cholesterol: 112mg | Sodium: 168mg | Potassium: 661mg | Sugar: 1g | Vitamin C: 1.6mg | Calcium: 11mg | Iron: 3.1mg

Air Fryer Plantain Chips

Prep Time: 5 Mins

Cook Time: 12 Mins

Total Time: 17 Mins

Ingredients

1 Green Plantain Evenly sliced

1 Tsp. Kosher Salt or to taste

1 Cup Water

Lemon or Lime Juice Optional

Instructions

Add the water and salt to a bowl. Stir. Set aside.

Peel the plantains.

Sliced the plantains in even slices. Best to use a mandolin.

Add the plantain slices to the salted water, let soak for about 5-10 minutes.

Transfer to the air fryer. Spray with olive oil, cook for 12 minutes, shaking and spraying with oil in between cooking. Increase the time for desired crispiness. Sprinkle with lemon or lime juice (optional). Enjoy!

Nutrition Value

Calories: 537kcal, Carbohydrates: 141g, Protein: 3g, Fat: 2g, Sodium: 1147mg, Potassium: 2163mg, Fiber: 8g, Sugar: 78g, Vitamin A: 120IU, Vitamin C: 165mg, Calcium: 10mg, Iron: 18mg

Easy Green Bean Fries (Keto + Low Carb)

Prep Time: 15 MINUTES

Total Time: 15 MINUTES

Ingredients

1 pound of green beans, ends trimmed if needed

1 egg

1 tablespoon of low-carb ranch dressing, jalapeño ranch dressing, or mayonnaise

1 cup almond flour

1/2 teaspoon garlic salt

1/2 teaspoon pepper

1/2 teaspoon garlic powder

1/2 cup parmesan cheese

Air Fryer Instructions:

Preheat your machine according to the directions at 390 degrees F.

When hot, add in as many green beans as you comfortably can without overcrowding.

Spray with cooking spray to help crisp.

Cook 5 minutes, shaking the basket halfway through cooking to move them around.

Nutrition Information

Calories: 143| Total Fat: 5.3g| Carbohydrates: 8.1g| Fiber: 2.5g| Sugar: 3.1g| Protein: 7g

Roasted Okra

Prep Time: 5 minutes

Cook Time: 15 minutes

Total Time: 20 minutes

Ingredients

1/2 pound small whole okra, per person

Salt to taste

Pepper to taste (or seasonings of choice)

Olive oil spray (optional, if needed to prevent sticking)

Instructions

First, start with the smallest okra you can find. Larger okra tends to be woody, which wouldn't work in this recipe.

Wash the okra. Trim off any excess stems, but do not cut into the okra pod itself.

Preheat the oven to 450 F. Spray a shallow baking dish with olive oil, if necessary, add okra, and season to taste. Give the okra one quick (1/2 second) spray with olive oil and put them into the oven. Bake, stirring every 5 minutes until okra is browned on all sides, about 15 minutes. Serve hot out of the oven.

<u>Air Fryer Instructions</u>

Preheat a standard air fryer to 390F or a Breville Air to 425F. Toss the freshly washed okra with seasoning and spread it in a single layer in the air fryer basket. Begin air frying, checking after about 7 minutes. Air fry until the okra is browning on all sides.

Nutrition Facts

Fat: 0.2g, Sodium: 9mg, Carbohydrates: 16g, Fiber: 7g, Protein: 5g

Easy Air Fryer Green Beans

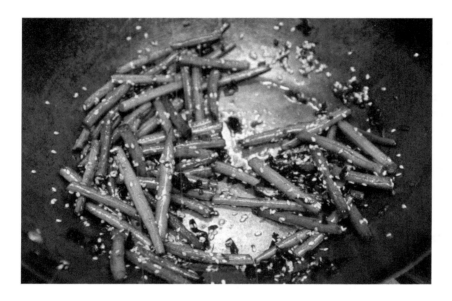

Prep Time: 2 mins

Cook Time: 6 mins

Total Time: 8 mins

Ingredients

1 lb (450g) green beans

Cooking spray

Salt

Instructions

Preheat the air fryer to 400 F / 200C.

Add the green beans to a bowl and spray with some low-calorie spray and the best salt ever and combine.

Place the beans into the air fryer basket and cook for 6-8 minutes, turning a couple of times during cooking so that they brown evenly.

Remove and serve topped with some extra salt and chopped herbs if you like.

Nutrition

Calories: 35kcal | Carbohydrates: 7g | Protein: 2g | Sodium: 6mg | Potassium: 239mg | Fiber: 3g | Sugar: 3g | Vitamin A: 785IU | Vitamin C: 13.9mg | Calcium: 42mg | Iron: 1.2mg

Air Fryer Caramelized Stone Fruit

Prep Time: 3 minutes

Cook Time: 15 minutes

Total Time: 15 minutes

Ingredients

1 lbs / 2-3 stone fruits such as peaches, nectarines, plums, or apricots

1 tbsp maple syrup

1/2 tbsp coconut sugar

1/4 tsp cinnamon, optional

Pinch of salt, optional

Instructions

Prepare Air Fryer: Cut a sheet of parchment paper that will fit the floor of your air fryer basket and then place it inside the basket.

Prepare Fruit: Slice the stone fruit down the middle and remove the seed. Then brush some maple syrup on the flesh and sprinkle with some coconut sugar. Add in a pinch of cinnamon and salt if desired.

Air Fry: Place the stone fruit in the air fryer basket and air fry at 350 for 15 minutes or until caramelized.

Nutrition Value

Calories: 124 Sugar: 27.8g| Sodium: 1.2mg| Fat: 0.6g| Unsaturated Fat: 0.4g| Carbohydrates: 31.1g| Fiber: 3.4g| Protein: 2.1g

Spinach Apple Smoothie

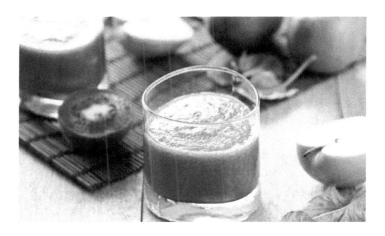

Prep Time: 5 Minutes

Total Time: 5 Minutes

Ingredients

1 Banana, sliced

½ Apple, finely diced

1 cup Baby Spinach Leaves

½ cup Filtered Water

1 tbsp Chia Seeds

½ Lime, juiced

Instructions

Put all ingredients in a high-performance blender and blend for 30-60 seconds until smooth.

Pour, serve and enjoy!

Nutrition Information:

Calories: 256| Total Fat: 5g| Saturated Fat: 1g| Trans Fat: 0g| Unsaturated Fat: 4g| Cholesterol: 0mg| Sodium: 135mg| Carbohydrates: 53g| Fiber: 14g| Sugar: 25g| Protein: 9g

Green Apple Lemon Cucumber Ginger Smoothie

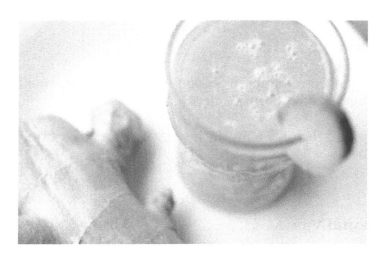

Prep Time: 10 Mins

Total Time: 10 Mins

Ingredients

3/4 cup coconut water, or water

2 green apples, cored and quartered

1/4 English cucumber, chopped

1/2 bunch flat-leaf parsley, leaves only, chopped

1 slice piece ginger, 1 inch thick

1 medium lemon, peeled and seeded

1 cup ice cubes

Instructions

Place all the Ingredients in a good quality blender, starting with the liquids and blend until smooth.

Optional, run through a mesh sieve if you don't like it pulpy. Pour into 2 glasses with ice.
Pour into 2 glasses with ice.

Nutritional Value

Calories: 110kcal| Carbohydrates: 30.5g| Protein: 2g| Fat: 0.5g| Sodium: 20mg| Fiber: 6.5g| Sugar: 18g

Blueberry Smoothie Recipe With Fresh Mint

Prep Time: 5 minutes

Total Time: 5 minutes

Ingredients

1 cup blueberries

1 cup Greek yogurt

2 tablespoons honey

1/2 cup water

10 mint leaves

Instructions

Combine all ingredients in the blender. Puree until smooth.

Serve immediately.

Nutrition Value

Calories: 193kcal | Carbohydrates: 34.2g | Protein: 11.6g | Fat: 2.5g | Saturated Fat: 1.6g | Cholesterol: 5mg | Sodium: 44mg | Fiber: 3.7g | Sugar: 28.5g

Kale Smoothie

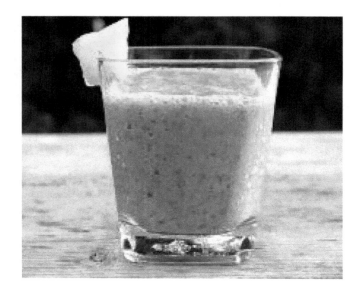

Prep Time: 5 Minutes

Cook Time: 5 Minutes

Total Time: 10 Minutes

Ingredients

3 cups kale chopped

1 cup plain yogurt or vanilla yogurt

1 ¼ cup orange juice or as needed

2 bananas frozen

1 cup frozen fruit of your choice I prefer pineapple or strawberry.

2 teaspoons honey or preferred sweetener

Instructions

Blend kale, yogurt, and orange juice until smooth.

Add remaining ingredients and blend until smooth.

Divide over two glasses and serve immediately.

Nutrition Information

Calories: 388| Carbohydrates: 81g| Protein: 11g| Fat: 6g| Saturated Fat: 3g| Cholesterol: 16mg| Sodium: 103mg| Potassium: 1521mg| Fiber: 5g| Sugar: 52g| Vitamin C: 212mg| Calcium: 328mg| Iron: 2mg

Dairy-Free Green Protein Smoothie

Prep Time: 4 Minutes

Blend Time: 1 Minute

Total Time: 5 Minutes

Ingredients

1 cup unsweetened almond milk

1 scoop vanilla protein powder, Use your favorite brand

1 medium banana, cut into chunks, and frozen

2 cups baby spinach

Instructions

Add almond milk, protein powder, banana chunks, and spinach into the blender.

Blend for a full minute, or until the spinach is broken down and the smoothie is smooth with no banana or spinach chunks.

Nutrition Information

Calories: 265| Total Fat: 7g| Saturated Fat: 0g| Trans Fat: 0g| Unsaturated Fat: 0g| Cholesterol: 40mg| Sodium: 261mg| Carbohydrates: 40g| Fiber: 13g| Sugar: 14g| Protein: 27g

Detox And Immune Boosting Smoothie

Prep Time: 5 mins

Cook Time: 2 mins

Total Time: 7 mins

Ingredients

1 apple

1 orange

1 kiwi,

1 medium carrot (or 3-4 baby carrots)

1 strawberry,

1 tbs apple cider vinegar,

½ cup of water

And optional: 3-4 cubes of ice.

Instructions

Wash fresh produce. Add to your blender: 1 Apple, 1 orange 1 kiwi, 1 medium Carrot (or 3-4 baby carrots) 1 strawberry, 1 TBS Apple cider vinegar, ½ cup of water, and optional: 3-4 cubes of ice.

Blend it all for 1-2 minutes depending on how powerful your blender is and enjoy right away.

Delicious first thing in the morning and great for any time during the day.

Nutritional Value

Calories: 201kcal | Carbohydrates: 1g | Protein: 28g | Fat: 29g | Saturated Fat: 14g | Cholesterol: 112mg | Sodium: 168mg | Potassium: 661mg | Sugar: 1g | Vitamin C: 16mg | Calcium: 11mg | Iron: 3.1mg

Green Mango Superfood Smoothie

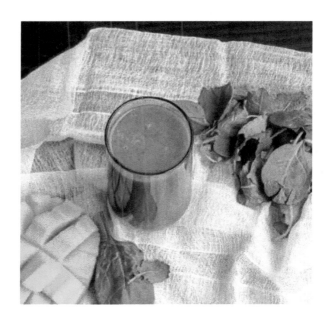

Prep Time: 5 mins

Total Time: 5 mins

Ingredients

1 cup spinach packed

1 1/4 cups almond milk

1.5 cups frozen ripe mango chunks

1 teaspoon ground flax

1 tablespoon chia seeds

1/8 teaspoon almond extract

Instructions

Combine the spinach and almond milk in a blender and blend until smooth.

Add the mango chunks, flax, chia seeds, and almond extract. Blend again until smooth.

Nutrition Value

Calories: 289kcal | Carbohydrates: 41g | Protein: 7g | Fat: 9g | Sodium: 474mg | Fiber: 12g | Sugar: 29g

Anti-Inflammatory Turmeric Smoothie With Pineapple

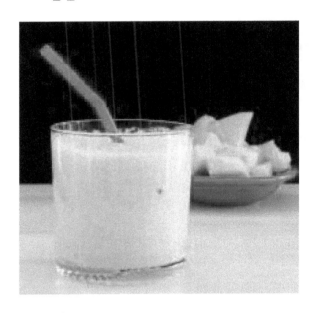

Prep Time: 10 mins

Total Time: 10 mins

Ingredients

1 1/4 cups almond milk

1 cup kale or spinach packed

1/4 teaspoon turmeric

1 pinch black pepper

1 tablespoon chia seeds

1 1/2 cups pineapple chunks frozen

Instructions

Combine the first 5 ingredients in a blender and blend until smooth.

Add the pineapple chunks and blend again until completely smooth.

Nutrition Value

Calories: 305kcal | Carbohydrates: 49g | Protein: 5g | Fat: 7g | Saturated Fat: 1g | Sodium: 456mg | Fiber: 14g | Sugar: 36g

Triple Berry Kiwi Smoothie.

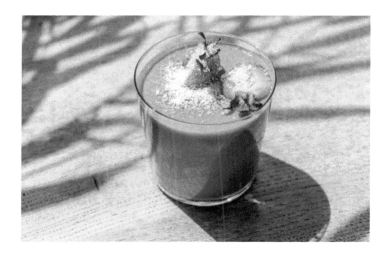

Prep Time: 10 minutes

Total Time: 10 minutes

Ingredients

1 cup frozen strawberries

3/4 cup frozen raspberries

1/2 cup frozen blueberries

2 kiwifruit peeled and sliced

1 cup orange juice

Instructions

Place the frozen berries in the blender and let them thaw for about 10 minutes.

Add the kiwifruit and the orange juice and blend on high until smooth.

Top with more kiwi or berries if desired.

Nutrition Facts

Fat: 2g, Sodium: 11mg, Potassium: 1477mg, Carbohydrates: 85g, Fiber: 16g, Sugar: 55g, Protein: 6g, Vitamin: C 408.1mg, Calcium: 135mg, Iron: 2.5mg

Immunity Boosting Orange Smoothie

Prep Time: 5 mins

Total Time: 5 mins

Ingredients

1 large orange (peeled)

½ medium banana

1 cup frozen mango pieces

½ cup almond milk

¼ teaspoon vanilla extract

Instructions

Place all Ingredients in a blender and blend until smooth. Serve immediately.

Nutrition Value

Calories: 233kcal | Carbohydrates: 54g | Protein: 3g | Fat: 2g | Sodium: 164mg | Potassium: 725mg | Fiber: 7g | Sugar: 42g | Vitamin C: 134.9mg | Calcium: 221mg | Iron: 0.3mg

Immune Boosting Multi-Colored Beet Smoothies

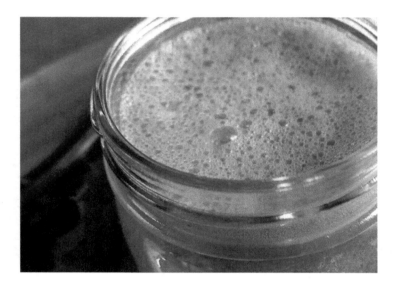

Prep Time: 10 mins

Total Time: 10 mins

Ingredients

2 small or 1 big beet – red yellow, or both – peeled and cut into cubes

1 (14 oz.) can of whole coconut milk

1 frozen banana in small pieces

12-14 red seedless grapes

1 tablespoon lime juice freshly squeezed

1 cup baby spinach or kale rinsed (optional)

1 cup ice

Instructions

Place beets, coconut milk, banana, grapes, lime juice, spinach (or kale), and ice in a blender. Blend until smooth. Divide it in between 2 glasses and serve immediately.

Nutrition Value

Calories: 587kcal | Carbohydrates: 41g | Protein: 8g | Fat: 48g | Saturated Fat: 42g | Sodium: 114mg | Potassium: 1226mg | Fiber: 9g | Sugar: 24g | Vitamin A: 3411IU | Vitamin C: 58mg | Calcium: 95mg | Iron: 5mg

Kale Pineapple Smoothie

Prep Time: 5 mins

Cook Time: 5 mins

Total Time: 10 mins

Ingredients

2 cups kale rinsed, stems removed, and coarsely chopped

1 ½ cups fresh pineapple cubed

1 tablespoon chia seeds

1 ripe banana peeled and cut into small chunks

1 ½ cups unsweetened almond milk

Maple syrup - optional

1 ½ cups ice

Instructions

Place all ingredients in a blender. Blend until fully mixed and smooth.

Taste for sweetness and add in maple syrup if you think it is necessary.

Serve immediately.

Nutrition Value

Calories: 101kcal | Carbohydrates: 19g | Protein: 3g | Fat: 3g |
Saturated Fat: 1g | Sodium: 140mg | Potassium: 350mg | Fiber:
3g | Sugar: 10g | Vitamin C: 72mg | Calcium: 192mg | Iron: 1mg

Carrot-Ginger Citrus Immune Boosting Smoothie

Prep Time: 5 minutes

Cook Time :1 minute

Total Time: 6 minutes

Ingredients

1 Navel or Cara Cara Orange or three small oranges such as mandarin or satsuma, peeled

1 Thin Slice of Lemon, leave the skin on

2 Medium Carrots chopped

1 Banana sliced into chunks, frozen is preferred for extra creamy and chill

1 inch (2.5cm) knob of Fresh Ginger make this 1 1/2" if you love ginger, leave the skin on

3 Tbs Hemp Hearts or a small handful of preferred nuts such as cashews

1/2 tsp Ground Turmeric

1 C (235g) Water

Instructions

Into the pitcher of a high-speed blender (I use Vitamix) add the orange(s), lemon, carrots, banana, ginger, hemp hearts, turmeric, and water. Start on low and increase speed up to high until all the ingredients are smooth. About 45 seconds. Pour into a glass and top with a sprinkle hemp hearts.

Nutrition Value

Calories: 251kcal | Carbohydrates: 32g | Protein: 10g | Fat: 11g | Saturated Fat: 1g | Sodium: 51mg | Potassium: 541mg | Fiber: 6g | Sugar: 16g | Vitamin C: 57mg | Calcium: 82mg | Iron: 4mg

Green Smoothie Basics

Total Time: 15 mins

Ingredients

1 cup milk or juice

1 cup spinach or kale

½ cup banana or ½ cup plain yogurt

1 cup fruit today that's 1 kiwi and 1 pear

1 Tbsp optional superfood topping chia, flax, or hemp seeds

1 tsp optional flavor enhancer cinnamon, vanilla, honey

Instructions

Combine liquid and greens in a blender until smooth. Add the rest of your ingredients and continue blending until smooth. Serve immediately.

Nutrition

Calories: 210cal | Carbohydrates: 42g | Protein: 6g | Fat: 3g | Saturated Fat: 1g | Cholesterol: 5mg | Sodium: 71mg | Potassium: 591mg | Fiber: 5g | Sugar: 29g | Vitamin C: 11.7mg | Calcium: 206mg | Iron: 1.4mg

Skinny Green Tropical Smoothie

Prep Time: 5 Mins

Total Time: 5 Mins

Ingredients

3/4 cup light coconut milk

6 oz fat-free Greek yogurt

3/4 cup fresh pineapple, cubed

1 ripe medium banana

1 cup spinach

2 tbsp sweetened shredded coconut

1 1/4 cups ice

Instructions

Put everything into the blender and blend until smooth.

Nutritional Value

Serving: 1 3/4 cups| Calories: 228kcal| Carbohydrates: 30.2g| Protein: 10.2g| Fat: 7.7g| Saturated Fat: 0.2g| Sodium: 70.5mg| Fiber: 3.9g| Sugar: 19.4g

Superfood Pb Banana And Cacao Green Smoothie

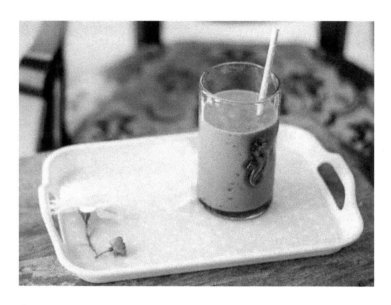

Prep Time: 5 Mins

Total Time: 5 Mins

Ingredients

3/4 cup unsweetened vanilla almond milk, I used Almond Breeze

1 loose cup baby spinach

2 teaspoons peanut butter

1/2 frozen ripe banana

1/3 oz heaping tablespoon cacao nibs (I used Navitas)

1 cup ice

Optional a few drops liquid stevia

Instructions

Combine all the ingredients in a blender and blend until smooth.

Nutritional Value

Serving: 1smoothie| Calories: 188kcal| Carbohydrates: 21g| Protein: 6g| Fat: 11.5g| Saturated Fat: 3.5g| Sodium: 210mg| Fiber: 6.5g| Sugar: 8.5g

Cucumber, Parsley, Pineapple, And Lemon Smoothie

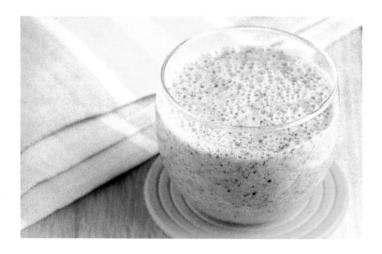

Prep Time: 10 Mins

Total Time: 10 Mins

Ingredients

3/4 cup coconut water, or water

1/2 english cucumber, chopped

1 bunch flat-leaf parsley, leaves only, chopped

2 medium lemons, peeled and seeded

2 cups fresh pineapple, frozen

5 drops liquid stevia, optional

Fresh ginger, optional

Instructions

Place all the Ingredients in a large blender and blast on high for 1 minute, until smooth and creamy.

Divide into two cups.

Nutritional Value

Calories: 118kcal| Carbohydrates: 31g| Protein: 2g| Sodium: 24mg| Fiber: 5g| Sugar: 18g

Extra Veggies Green Smoothie

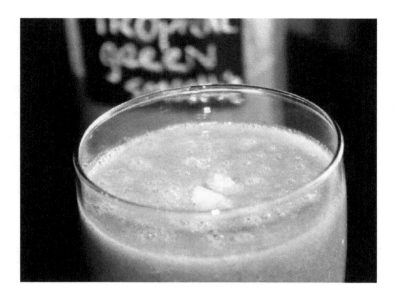

Prep Time: 5 mins

Total Time: 5 mins

Ingredients

½ banana (preferably frozen)

½ cup kale or spinach

½ zucchini, peeled and chopped

½ avocado

2 Tbsp chia seeds

2 Tbsp flax seeds

1 cup unsweetened almond milk

Instructions

Add everything to a blender, and blend on the highest speed for at least 20 seconds until completely smooth.

Nutritional Value

Saturated Fat 2.9g, Polyunsaturated Fat 12.1g, Monounsaturated Fat 10.2g, Sodium 203.7mg, Total Carbohydrate 36.8g, Dietary Fiber 19.3g, Sugars 7.8g, Protein 10.9g

Spinach Apple Smoothie

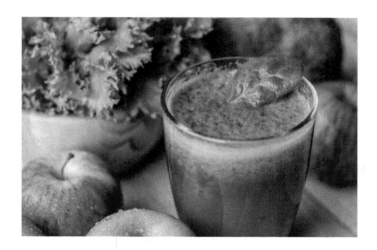

Prep Time: 5 Minutes

Total Time: 5 Minutes

Ingredients

1 Banana, sliced

½ Apple, finely diced

1 cup Baby Spinach Leaves

½ cup Filtered Water

1 tbsp Chia Seeds

½ Lime, juiced

Instructions

Put all ingredients in a high-performance blender and blend for 30-60 seconds until smooth.

Pour, serve and enjoy!

NUTRITION INFORMATION

Calories: 256| Total Fat: 5g| Saturated Fat: 1g| Unsaturated Fat: 4g| Sodium: 135mg| Carbohydrates: 53g| Fiber: 14g| Sugar: 25g| Protein: 9g

Green Goddess Smoothie

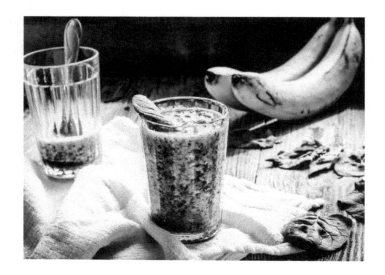

Prep Time: 5 minutes

Total Time: 5 minutes

Ingredients

2 green apples

1 banana (frozen preferred)

2 cups kale or spinach

4 Tablespoons peanut butter

2 Tablespoons flaxseeds

2 Tablespoons maple syrup

2 cups almond milk

Instructions

Place all ingredients in a blender and blend until smooth.

Nutrition

Calories: 510kcal | Carbohydrates: 68g | Protein: 15g | Fat: 24g | Saturated Fat: 3g | Sodium: 504mg | Potassium: 1068mg | Fiber: 11g | Sugar: 41g | Vitamin C: 93.9mg | Calcium: 472mg | Iron: 2.5mg

Green Mango Superfood Smoothie

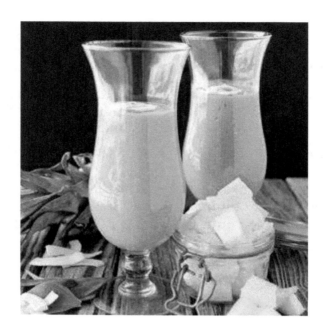

Prep Time: 5 mins

Total Time: 5 mins

Ingredients

1 cup spinach packed

1 1/4 cups almond milk

1.5 cups frozen ripe mango chunks

1 teaspoon ground flax

1 tablespoon chia seeds

1/8 teaspoon almond extract

Instructions

Combine the spinach and almond milk in a blender and blend until smooth.

Add the mango chunks, flax, chia seeds, and almond extract. Blend again until smooth.

Nutrition Value

Calories: 289kcal | Carbohydrates: 41g | Protein: 7g | Fat: 9g | Sodium: 474mg | Fiber: 12g | Sugar: 29g

Simple Spinach Green Smoothie

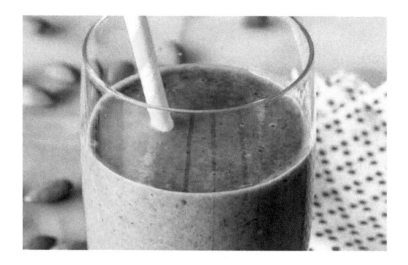

Prep Time: 1 minute

Cook Time: 4 minutes

Total Time: 5 minutes

Ingredients

2 cups fresh spinach

1 banana fresh or frozen, frozen is best

1 cup almond milk

1 scoop of protein powder

1 tsp lime juice

Instructions

Add spinach, almond milk, banana, protein powder, lime juice into a blender.

Blend until creamy.

Pour into a glass garnish with mint and lime, enjoy!

Nutrition Value

Calories: 144kcal | Carbohydrates: 20g | Protein: 15g | Fat: 2g | Polyunsaturated Fat: 1g | Cholesterol: 3mg | Sodium: 54mg | Fiber: 3g | Sugar: 11g

Healthy And Easy Green Smoothie

Prep Time: 15 Minutes

Ingredients

1/2 cup frozen fruit (any kind you like!)

1 medium banana

1 cup low-fat yogurt (any kind you like!)

A handful of baby spinach

1 tbsp. honey (optional)

Splash of juice or milk (optional - depending on how thick you like it)

Instructions

Add all Ingredients to a blender. Cover and blend until smooth.

Serve!

Nutrition Information:

Calories: 296| Total Fat: 4g| Saturated Fat: 3g| Cholesterol: 15mg| Sodium: 177mg| Fiber: 4g| Sugar: 32g| Protein: 15g

Double Green Smoothie

Active Time: 5 Mins

Total Time: 5 Mins

Ingredients

1 cup baby spinach (about 1 ounce) 1 Roasted Golden Beet, chopped 1/2 fresh or frozen ripe banana 1/2 cup brewed green tea, chilled 1/4 cup unsweetened almond milk 1 1/2 tablespoons flaxseed meal

Nutritional Information

Calories: 196| Fat: 7g| Sat Fat: 1g| Unsatfat: 5g| Protein: 6g| Carbohydrate: 29g| Fiber: 9g| Sugars: 15g| Sodium: 274mg

Green Smoothie Recipe

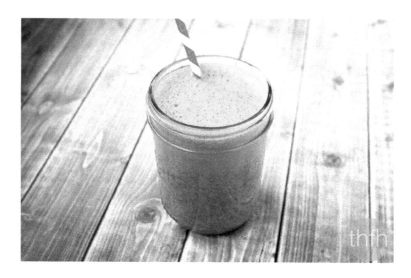

Prep Time: 5 Minutes

Total Time: 5 Minutes

Ingredients

½ cup yogurt plain or Greek

2 cups kale chopped

1 banana

1 cup pineapple chopped

1 tablespoon flax seeds

1 cup milk

Honey to taste optional

Instructions

Add yogurt, kale, banana, pineapple, flax seeds, and milk to the blender.

Blend until smooth.

Add honey to taste if desired. Serve immediately.

Nutrition Information

Calories: 240| Carbohydrates: 40g| Protein: 10g| Fat: 6g| Saturated Fat: 2g| Cholesterol: 13mg| Sodium: 108mg| Potassium: 942mg| Fiber: 4g| Sugar: 24g| Vitamin C: 125mg| Calcium: 346mg| Iron: 1.7mg

Super Green Smoothie

Prep Time: 2 min

Cook Time: 1 min

Ready In : 3 min

Ingredients

Blender Version

Makes about 1½–2 cups (375–500mL)

Average Yield: 1½ cups (374 mL)

½ cup (125 mL) apple juice

1 cup (250 mL) torn kale leaves

1 banana, quartered

Smoothie Cup Version

½ avocado, cut in half

½ cup (125 mL) ice

½ cup (125 mL) ice

½ cup (125 mL) torn kale leaves

1 banana, quartered

½ avocado, cut in half

½ cup (125 mL) apple juice

Direction

Add all the ingredients, in the order listed, to the Deluxe Cooking Blender.

Replace and lock the lid. Turn the wheel to select the SMOOTHIE setting; press the wheel to start.

Attached the adapter to the base of the Deluxe Cooking Blender. Fill the smoothie cup with the ingredients, in the order listed; do not fill past the max fill line. When the sleeve is on the cup, make sure it's dry and secure.

Screw blade lid clockwise onto the cup to secure. Turn the cup upside down and align the cup notches with the adapter slots; turn counterclockwise and secure. Turn the wheel to select the SMOOTHIE setting; press the wheel to start.

Directions

Garnish as desired and enjoy!

Nutrients Value

Calories: 320| Total Fat: 15 G| Saturated Fat: 2.5g| Sodium: 20 Mg, Carbohydrate: 50g| Fiber: 10g| Total Sugars: 28g| Protein: 4 G

Cool Cucumber Green Smoothie

Prep Time: 10 minutes

Cook Time: 0 minutes

Total: 10 minutes

Ingredients

1/2 c. almond milk

1/2 c. apple juice or orange juice

1/2 cucumber

1/2 banana

1/2 c. frozen strawberries

1/2 c. pineapple

2 handfuls of leafy greens I did a combo of spinach, kale, and chard

Instructions

Add liquids to the blender first, then add all the remaining Ingredients.

Blend until smooth.

Makes one serving (250 calories)

Alternatives- eliminate juice to make it 65 calories less, or add 1 Tbsp raw peanut butter for protein (add 90 calories).

Nutrition Value

Calories: 251kcal | Carbohydrates: 58g | Protein: 5g | Fat: 3g | Saturated Fat: 1g | Sodium: 185mg | Potassium: 982mg | Fiber: 7g | Sugar: 38g | Vitamin C: 155.7mg | Calcium: 208mg | Iron: 1.7mg

Morning Green Smoothie

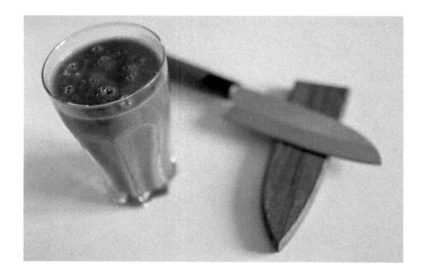

Prep Time: 3 minutes

Cook Time: 1 minute

Ingredients

1 1/2 cups Water

1 cup Spinach

1/3 cup Pineapple frozen

1/3 cup Mango Frozen

1 Cara Cara Orange peeled

1/2 Banana frozen

1 tablespoon Chia Seeds

1 cup Ice

Instructions

Arrange the Ingredients in your blender as shown, from the water first to the ice last.

Blend until smoothie and pour into your favorite glasses to enjoy.

Nutrition Value

Calories: 80kcal | Carbohydrates: 17g | Protein: 2g | Fat: 1g | Saturated Fat: 1g | Sodium: 16mg | Potassium: 272mg | Fiber: 4g | Sugar: 11g | Vitamin C: 43mg | Calcium: 56mg | Iron: 1mg

Air Fryer Green Beans With Lemon (Healthy & Vegan!)

Prep Time: 5 Minutes

Cook Time: 20 Minutes

Total Time: 25 Minutes

Ingredients

2 lbs green beans, washed & trimmed

2 tablespoon olive oil

¾ teaspoon salt

2 tablespoons lemon juice

Instructions

Preheat the air fryer to 400 degrees for 5 minutes.

In a large bowl, toss the beans in the olive oil until they are evenly covered with oil.

Sprinkle the beans with ½ teaspoon salt and toss further until the salt evenly covers all the beans.

Add the beans to the air fryer basket and air fry for 17-19 minutes, shaking the beans every 4 minutes, or until the beans are blistered and browning around the edges,

Pour the beans into a large serving bowl and squeeze or pour the lemon juice over the beans. Toss the beans until they're covered with the lemon juice and season with up to an extra ¼ teaspoon salt to taste.

Nutrition Information

Calories: 70, Total Fat: 4g, Saturated Fat: 1g, Unsaturated Fat: 3g, Sodium: 200mg, Carbohydrates: 9g, Fiber: 4g, Sugar: 4g, Protein: 2g

Asian-Inspired Air Fryer Green Beans

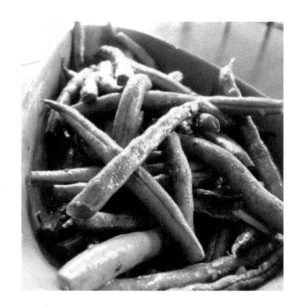

Prep Time: 5 minutes

Cook Time: 10 minutes

Total Time: 15 minutes

Ingredients

8 ounces fresh green beans

1 Tablespoon tamari

1 teaspoon sesame oil

Instructions

Break off the ends of the green beans, then snap them in half.

Place the green beans in a resealable plastic bag or a container with a lid. Add the tamari and sesame oil and shake to coat.

Put the green beans in the basket of your air fryer. Cook at 390 or 400 degrees (depending on your air fryer model) for 10 minutes, tossing halfway through.

Nutrition Value

Calories: 58kcal | Carbohydrates: 8g | Protein: 3g | Fat: 2g | Sodium: 509mg | Potassium: 258mg | Fiber: 3g | Sugar: 3g | Vitamin C: 13.9mg | Calcium: 42mg | Iron: 1.4mg

Green Pina Colada Smoothie With Spinach And Mango

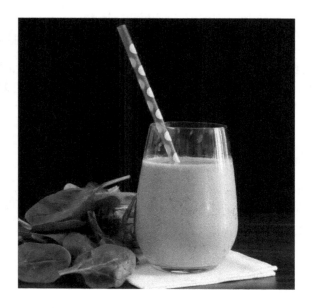

Prep Time: 5 minutes

Total Time: 5 minutes

Ingredients

2 Tablespoons cream of coconut or coconut milk

2 handfuls of baby spinach

1 cup frozen mango cut-up

1/2 cup fresh pineapple

1/2 frozen banana sliced

1/2 avocado

1 Tablespoon lemon juice

Scoop vanilla protein powder

Instructions

Place all ingredients in a blender and blend until smooth.

Nutrition Value

Calories: 651kcal | Carbohydrates: 94g | Protein: 25g | Fat: 24g | Saturated Fat: 9g | Cholesterol: 62mg | Sodium: 154mg | Potassium: 1524mg | Fiber: 15g | Sugar: 66g | Vitamin C: 137mg | Calcium: 254mg | Iron: 3mg

Hemp And Greens Smoothie

Prep Time: 5 mins

Ingredients

1½ cups fresh spinach leaves, packed

¼ cup hulled hemp seeds

1 cup chilled coconut water, or more to thin

1-inch knob ginger, peeled

½ cup frozen banana slices

1 cup frozen pineapple chunks

Instructions

Add all ingredients (in order) to a blender. Puree until smooth. This yields a hearty smoothie for 1 or two small smoothies!

Nutrition Value

Calories: 229kcal | Carbohydrates: 21g | Protein: 11g | Fat: 11g | Saturated Fat: 1g | Sodium: 145mg | Potassium: 604mg | Fiber: 4g | Sugar: 11g | Vitamin C: 32.2mg | Calcium: 91mg | Iron: 4.6mg

Air Fryer Green Beans

Prep Time: 10 minutes

Cook Time: 10 minutes

Total Time: 20 minutes

Ingredients

24 ounces fresh green beans - trimmed

2 cups sliced button mushrooms

1 fresh lemon - juiced

1 tablespoon garlic powder

¾ teaspoon ground sage

1 teaspoon onion powder

¾ teaspoon salt

¾ teaspoon black pepper

Spray oil

⅓ cup french fried onions - for garnish, optional

Instructions

In a large bowl, toss together the green beans, mushrooms, lemon juice, garlic powder, sage, onion powder, salt, and pepper. Transfer the mixture to your air fryer basket, then use spray oil to coat, shaking well.

Air fry at 400° F for 10-12 minutes, shaking every 2-3 minutes.

Serve topped with french fried onions, if you're using them.

Nutrition Value

Calories: 65kcal

Air Fryer Garlic Roasted Green Beans

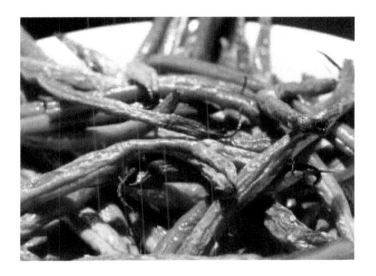

Prep Time: 2 minutes

Cook Time: 8 minutes

Total Time: 10 minutes

Ingredients

3/4-1 pound fresh green beans (trimmed)

1 tablespoon olive oil

1 teaspoon garlic powder

Salt and pepper to taste

Instructions

Drizzle the olive oil over the green beans. Sprinkle the seasonings throughout. Toss to coat.

Place the green beans in the air fryer basket.

Cook the green beans for 7-8 minutes at 370 degrees. Toss the basket halfway through the total cook time.

Remove the green beans and serve.

Nutrition Value

Calories: 45kcal | Carbohydrates: 3g | Protein: 1g | Fat: 3g

Tropical Mango & Arugula Smoothie

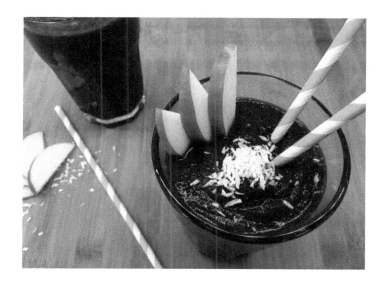

Prep Time: 5 minutes

Total Time: 5 minutes

Ingredients

Mango & Arugula Smoothie:

¾ cup coconut water

2 cups arugula

½ avocado

½ lime, zest & juice

1 cup frozen mango

¼ cup coconut shreds

Instructions

Add all ingredients to a blender and blend until smooth.

Serve with desired toppings and enjoy!

Yields 2 servings mango & arugula smoothie.

Nutrition Value

Calories: 220| Sugar: 17g| Fat: 18g| Carbohydrates: 25g| Fiber: 7g| Protein: 3g

Matcha Smoothie

Prep Time: 5 minutes

Total Time: 5 minutes

Ingredients

2 ripe bananas frozen

1 cup coconut milk

2 tsp matcha powder

1 cup spinach, frozen if desired

¼ cup frozen pineapple

Instructions

Add all ingredients to a blender and blend until smooth.

Pour into a glass, serve, and enjoy!

I like to top mine with coconut shreds and some toasted coconut flakes, but you can use any toppings you prefer!

Nutrition

Calories:301 | Sugar:9g | Fat:27g |Carbohydrates:31g |Fiber: 5g | Protein: 5g

Green Smoothie

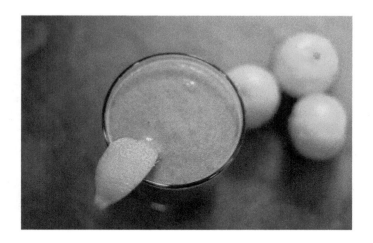

Prep Time: 5 Mins

Total Time: 5 Mins

Ingredients

1 ½ cups packed kale

⅔ cup orange juice or as needed

1 cup vanilla yogurt

1 banana

2 cups frozen pineapple

½ cup ice

Instructions

Blend kale and orange juice until smooth.

Add remaining ingredients and blend until thickened and creamy.

If your mixture is too thick, add orange juice as needed.

Nutrition Information

Calories: 301| Fat: 3g| Saturated Fat: 1g| Cholesterol: 6mg| Sodium: 106mg| Potassium: 1071mg| Carbohydrates: 65g| Fiber: 4g| Sugar: 47g| Protein: 10g|

Mango Avocado Smoothie

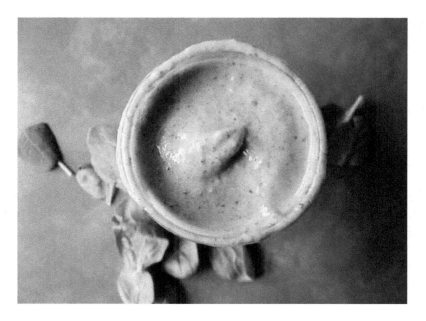

Prep Time: 5 mins

Total Time: 5 mins

Ingredients

2 cups spinach (either whole baby spinach or English spinach with the stalks removed)

2 cups coconut water

1 cup frozen mango

1 frozen banana

½ cup frozen avocado

2 tbsp almond butter

Instructions

Pop the spinach and coconut water into a high-speed blender and blend on high until well combined.

Add the other ingredients and blend until everything is well combined and smooth.

Serve, topping with granola, hemp seeds, or chia seeds (optional)

Nutrition Value

Calories: 156kcal | Carbohydrates: 21g | Protein: 4g | Fat: 8g | Saturated Fat: 1g | Sodium: 140mg | Potassium: 709mg | Fiber: 5g | Sugar: 13g | Vitamin A: 1899IU | Vitamin C: 27mg | Calcium: 76mg | Iron: 1mg

Lettuce Smoothie

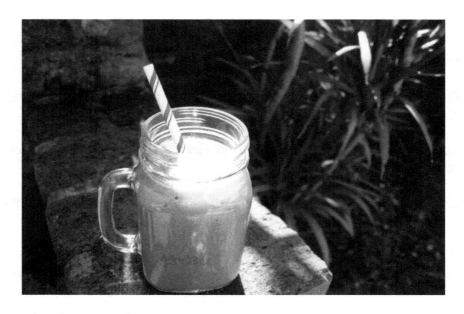

Prep Time: 5 minutes

Total Time: 5 minutes

Ingredients

2 cups chopped romaine lettuce

1 frozen banana

1/2 cup diced apple

1 and 1/2 cups almond milk

1 Tbsp. chia seeds

1 Tbsp. honey, if desired

Instructions

Add all of the ingredients into a blender. If you'd like a sweeter smoothie, add the honey, but if not, simply omit it.

Process until smooth.

Pour into glasses & enjoy.

Nutritional Facts

Calories: 168, Total Fat: 4.5g, Sodium: 145mg, Sugar:19.2, Vitamin A: 292Ug, Protein: 3.6g, Vitamin C: 8.4mg, Carbohydrtaes:31.5g

Glowing Green Smoothie Recipe

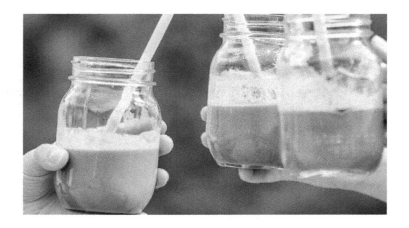

Prep Time: 5 mins

Ingredients

1/4 cup frozen pineapple chunks

1/4 cup frozen mango

1/2 banana

1/2 cup frozen or fresh baby spinach packed

1/2 cup water or milk of your choice

1 scoop truvani collagen (this is my favorite collagen)

Flax seeds

Instructions

Add pineapple chunks, mango, banana, spinach, water, and a scoop of Truvani Collagen into a blender.

Blend for 1-2 minutes, or until the smoothie has a smooth texture. Pour into a tall glass. Garnish with flax seed and enjoy!

Nutrition Value

Calories: 53kcal | Carbohydrates: 13g | Protein: 1g | Fat: 1g | Saturated Fat: 1g | Sodium: 7mg | Potassium: 211mg | Fiber: 2g | Sugar: 7g | Vitamin C: 5mg

Spinach Loquat Smoothie

Prep Time: 10 minutes

Total Time: 10 minutes

Ingredients

1 banana

4 loquats pitted

1 cup spinach

1 cup water

1/2 tbsp chia seeds

Instructions

Throw a banana, loquats, spinach leaves, and water in a blender.

Blend it up, pour in a glass (or a jar!), and top with chia seeds.

Nutrition Value

Calories: 151kcal | Carbohydrates: 36g | Protein: 2g | Fat: 1g | Sodium: 25mg | Potassium: 760mg |Fiber: 5g | Sugar: 14g | Vitamin A: 3865IU | Vitamin C: 18.7mg | Calcium: 53mg | Iron: 1.1mg

Keto Green Smoothie

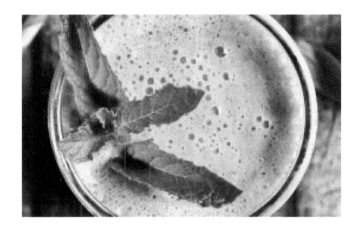

Prep Time: 5 Minutes

Additional Time: 5 Minutes

Total Time: 10 Minutes

Ingredients

2 cups baby spinach

1 1/2 cup unsweetened almond milk

1 cup frozen strawberry slices

½ cup frozen avocado chunks

2 tablespoons hemp seeds

3 drops Lakanto Monkfruit Extract, see note

Instructions

Add all ingredients to a blender and blend until smooth.

Divide between two glasses and drink immediately.

Nutrition Information

Calories: 148, Total Fat: 10g, Saturated Fat: 2g, Unsaturated Fat: 11g, Sodium: 172mg, Carbohydrates: 10g, Net Carbohydrates: 5g, Fiber: 5g, Protein: 6g

Tropical Green Smoothies

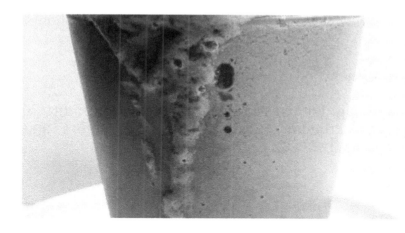

Prep Time: 15 mins

Ingredients

1 large handful of ice

2 cup orange juice or coconut water

1 cup pineapple

1 cup mango cored and peeled

1 pear cored, peel left intact

1 Granny Smith apple cored, peel left intact

1 large handful of spinach

1 large handful of kale

Instructions

Place items in a blender in the order listed. Blend until smooth. Keep covered with a lid in the refrigerator for up to 24 hours.

Nutrition Facts

Sodium: 102mg, Potassium: 411mg, Carbohydrates: 23g, Fiber: 4g, Sugar: 17g, Protein: 1g, Vitamin A: 435IU, Vitamin C: 33.5mg, Calcium: 36mg, Iron: 0.5mg

Cleansing Apple Avocado Smoothie

Prep Time: 5 Mins

Total Time: 5 Mins

Ingredients

1 cup plain unsweetened almond milk

4 cups loosely packed spinach that's about 2 large handfuls

1 medium avocado peeled and pitted

2 medium apples any kind you like, peel on, cored, and quartered (if not using a high-powered blender such as a Vitamix, cut into a rough dice)

1 medium banana cut into chunks and frozen

2 teaspoons honey or maple syrup plus additional to taste

1/2 teaspoon ground ginger or 1/4-inch knob of fresh ginger (if not using a high-power blender, mince the ginger first; use less than 1/2 teaspoon if you'd like a more subtle taste. This smoothie has some zip!)

A small handful of ice cubes

Optional additions: chia seeds flaxseed, protein powder, almond butter, or other nut butter of choice

Instructions

In the order listed, add the almond milk, spinach, avocado, apples, banana, honey, ginger, and ice to a high-powered blender.

Blend until smooth. Taste and adjust sweetness and spices as desired. Enjoy immediately.

Nutrition Facts

Calories: 306kcal, Carbohydrates: 15g, Protein: 4g, Fat: 13g, Saturated Fat: 2g, Sodium: 123mg, Fiber: 13g, Sugar: 30g

The Best Green Smoothie Recipe

Prep Time: 5 minutes

Total Time: 5 minutes

Ingredients

1 leaf kale - medium size

10 leaves dandelion greens

1 banana - frozen

1 green apple

1/2 cup orange juice - freshly squeezed (or 1 orange peel & seeds removed)

2 dates - pitted

1 tbsp hemp hearts

2 tsp apple cider vinegar

1/2 cup hemp milk or water + more to thin out to your liking 1 tsp spirulina powder

Instructions

Add all of the above smoothie ingredients except the apple cider vinegar to a powerful blender. Process until smooth and creamy to your liking. Add more plant milk, juice, or water If you'd like a thinner consistency. Balance the flavors to your taste with the apple cider vinegar and enjoy!

Nutrition Value

Calories: 212kcal | Carbohydrates: 41g | Protein: 6g | Fat: 4g | Sodium: 35mg | Potassium: 658mg |Fiber: 4g | Sugar: 26g | Vitamin A: 3605IU | Vitamin C: 76.2mg | Calcium: 75mg | Iron: 2.4mg

Lightning Source UK Ltd.
Milton Keynes UK
UKHW020653040521
383095UK00001B/71